Pain

Powerful Natural Remedies to Eliminate Aches, Pains and Inflammation Fast

Contents

Chapter 1. There are Pain Relief Alternatives

There is no longer a reason to deal with chronic pain. It doesn't matter if it's arthritis pain, knee pain, muscle pain, or back pain. You don't have to deal with it, and you don't have to turn to prescription medicine or over the counter drugs as a solution. There are natural pain relief remedies that can help you, and many of them are just as effective with less side effects.

There is no reason to tough it out. There is many ways that you can help other than just a pill. There are teas, smoothies, supplements, and even techniques that are known to help with even chronic pain. From neck aches to lower back pain and everything else, you can heal yourself and learn to cope with the pain without drugs.

Reasons to Try:

One reason people tend gravitate towards herbal remedies is that they are often a solution that's legal even if your doctor won't give you anything to help. Even if your doctor is giving you pain medication, usually you can only take it for so long before it becomes harmful or has harmful side effects.

With herbal remedies and natural remedies you have to worry about side effects a lot less. You always have to make sure that you don't have an allergy to an herbal remedy or natural treatment. Of course, you can get tested by your doctor, and you need to make sure your doctor is aware if you are taking herbal remedies.

Always Take Precaution:

It's important that you always take precaution when you are dealing with natural remedies. Natural techniques will not likely hurt you, but herbs can if you are allergic or if they interact with any over the counter or prescription medication that you're taking. If you want to be sure that you're not going to have a reaction, it is best that you talk to your doctor before adding it into anything.

You will need to check allergies, and you'll need to make sure that you proceed with caution. Always start out small in small doses, and know what you're taking before you take it. With herbal remedies you make yourself this is a little easier, but you also need to date everything.

Chapter 2. Pain Relief Teas to Help

Tea is soothing and is supposed to help relax your mind and calm your emotions. However, if you have the right tea it will help you with any physical pain that you're experiencing as well. Different teas will treat different types of chronic pain, but there is no reason that you should have to deal with pain so long as you have the right ingredients in your kitchen cabinet.

Tea #1 Inflammation & Pain Relief

Turmeric is anti-inflammatory, and it has curcumin in it that give sit the orange color as well as the anti-inflammatory effects. Turmeric I also known to help with the digestive system, and it has no toxic effects. It does not decrease your white blood cell count, it doesn't risk intestinal bleeding, and it doesn't risk ulcer formation unlike other drugs that are known for their anti-inflammatory effects.

Cayenne also has capsaicin, which is known for pain-reducing effects. It also has cardiovascular benefits, and it can prevent ulcers. Ginger has antioxidants as well as anti-inflammatory compounds. It can even help with nausea, and there's lemon which has vitamin C which will strengthen your immune system and keep painful swelling away. Black pepper is anti-spasmodic and anti-inflammatory as well. It's great at helping with muscle pain or even arthritis.

Ingredients:

1. 5 Cups Water, Filtered

2. ¼ Teaspoon Cayenne Powder

3. 2 Tablespoons Honey, Raw

4. 1 Lemon, Sliced

5. ½ Teaspoon Black Pepper, Ground

6. 1 Tablespoon Turmeric Powder

7. 1 Teaspoon Turmeric Powder

8. 2 Tablespoons Ginger, Grated

Direction:

1. Take a large saucepan, pouring the water into it. Squeeze the lemon into the water, and then add the slices into the pan. All remaining ingredients except the honey can be added as well, as you let it all come to a boil. Make sure that the spices are whisked in so that they thoroughly combine.

2. When it comes to a boil, remove it from heat. Leave it overnight in the refrigerator. Come back the next

morning, and straining it, adding in the raw honey to taste. Make sure it's stirred well before you drink.

Tea #2 Joint Pain Relief

Stinging nettle can cause discomfort if you brush up against it fresh, but the plant wen made into a tea can actually help to relieve discomfort. It especially helps with joint pain, and this is because it reduces inflammation. It can inhibit proteins that activate swelling along the joint, resulting in pain. It can even aid in kidney function and neutralize uric acid. It's cheap to get, and easy to use.

Ingredients:

1. 1 Teaspoon Nettle, Dried
2. 2 Cups Fresh Water
3. 2 Tablespoons Honey

Directions:

1. This simple nettle tea recipe is going to help with your joint pain, so start by boiling the water. When it comes to a boil, make sure that you add in the nettle leaves. Reduce it to a simmer.
2. Let simmer for five to six minutes. Remove from heat, and strain the nettle leaves out. Add in honey, and stir until it is completely mixed. Drink warm or chilled.

Tea #3 White Willow Bark Tea

You can take this tea two to three times daily, and it is slow to take effect. However, it does have long lasting effects. It helps with general pain relief, cramping, muscle spasms, and arthritis. It treats both pain and inflammation. You cannot take white willow bark if you are allergic to aspirin, and you should not take it with certain medication such as anticoagulants or an anti-platelet. Always tell your doctor that you plan to take white willow bark before you do so, which will help them to identify if you are taking anything that could interact with white willow bark tea. The cinnamon and honey is added for its taste, but cinnamon can also help with inflammation.

Ingredients:

1. 1 ½ Teaspoons White Willow Bark
2. 1 Cup Water
3. ½ Teaspoon Cinnamon, Ground
4. 1 Tablespoon Honey, Raw

Directions:

1. Boil the water with the white willow bark in it. Let it boil for four to five minutes, and then turn the heat off, letting the

white willow bark steep for twenty-five to thirty minutes.

2. Strain out the white willow bark, adding in the cinnamon and honey. Mix and drink hot or cold.

Tea #4 Tooth Pain Remedy

This can help with other pain as well, but this tea is mostly known for tooth pain. You can drink two to three cups a day, and that's why this recipe makes four to five. You can drink it warm or chilled. Cloves are the main ingredient to this pain relief remedy, and they're known to numb the pain. Of course ginger and cinnamon are both anti-inflammatory which will help as well. Use honey to sweeten, so you can feel free to use more or less as needed.

Ingredients:

1. 4 Tablespoons Cloves, Whole

2. 2 Cinnamon Sticks

3. 5 Cups Water

4. 3 Tablespoons Honey, Raw

5. 8 Slices Ginger Root, Fresh & Peeled

Directions:

1. Boil the water, and then steep all ingredients except the raw honey in it for twenty minutes.

2. Strain out, and then add in your honey. Chill or serve warm.

Tea #5 Ginger Tea

Ginger is anti-inflammatory, and it's great at any pain that is caused by swelling. This can help with arthritis and muscle pain. The cinnamon is also great for inflammation, and it's best that you take this remedy two to three times daily to get the best results.

Ingredients.

1. 2 Tablespoons Ginger, Grated & Fresh
2. 2 Teaspoon Honey, Raw
3. ½ Teaspoon Cinnamon, Ground

Directions:

1. Boil a cup of water, and then let the ginger and cinnamon steep for ten to twelve minutes.
2. Strain, and add in honey. Drink warm or chilled.

Chapter 3. Smoothie Recipes to Bring Relief

You can use smoothie recipes to get relief as well. You don't always have to have tea. Sometimes people want a sweet relief, and a smoothie can provide it for you. There are natural foods that are anti-inflammatory and help with pain, and often you can add these into your smoothie for the best results. Just make sure you're blender is clean and you're ready to go.

Smoothie #1 Muscle Pain Relief

Beet juice is a great way to relieve your muscle pain, and ginger and cinnamon are anti-inflammatory agents. The antioxidants in raspberries is also going to help you feel on top of your game. Make sure your beet juice doesn't have any added sugar, as it will interfere with the muscle relief. The honey is a natural way to sweeten your smoothie.

Ingredients:

1. 1 Cup Beet Juice, Chilled
2. 2 Tablespoons Honey
3. ½ Cup Raspberries, Frozen
4. 1 Teaspoon Ginger Powder
5. ½ Teaspoon Cinnamon, Ground

Directions:

1. Just blend until smooth, and then drink up.

Smoothie #2 Joint Pain Relief

You'll get two servings out of this joint pain relief smoothie, and the tart cherries are the main ingredient, but nutmeg helps with your joint pain as well. You'll be getting needed nutrients from the yogurt and strawberries, and the honey is a great way to naturally sweeten the mix. Add more honey if desired.

Ingredients:

1. 1 Cup Strawberries, frozen
2. 1 Cup Tart Cherries, Fresh & Pitted
3. ½ Cup Tart Cherry Juice, Chilled
4. 3 Tablespoons Orange Juice Concentrate
5. ½ Cup Vanilla Yogurt, Nonfat
6. 2 Tablespoons Honey
7. 1 Teaspoon Nutmeg, Ground

Directions:

1. All ingredients can be combined in your blender, and then blend until smooth.

Smoothie #3 Tropical Ginger & Turmeric Smoothie

A lot of chronic pain is caused by inflammation, and when you make sure that your smoothie is anti-inflammatory, then you're likely to help with your chronic pain. It can also help to brighten your day with this tropical, tasty smoothie.

Ingredients:

1. 1 Teaspoon Ginger, Ground
2. ½ Teaspoon Turmeric Powder
3. ½ Cup Pineapple, Chunked
4. ½ Cup Mango, Cubed & Frozen
5. ½ Cup Coconut Milk, Unsweetened & Chilled
6. 1 Teaspoon Honey, Raw

Directions:

1. Mix all ingredients together, and then blend until smooth. Add ice if needed to thicken.

Smoothie #4 A Boosted Blast

If you're looking for quick pain relief, the cinnamon and ginger will help. Blueberries help to boost your immune system with its antioxidants, and rosemary is also known to help with chronic pain relief. You have to add it in on a more regular basis, but it will help to relieve pain quickly. It even helps to improve circulation.

Ingredients:

1. 1 Cup Coconut Milk, Sweetened
2. 1 Teaspoon Honey, Raw
3. 2 Teaspoons Cinnamon, Ground
4. ½ Teaspoon Ginger
5. 1 Cup Blueberries, Frozen

6. 2 Teaspoons Rosemary, Ground

Directions:

1. Just mix everything together and blend
    until it is completely smooth.

Smoothie #5 Spicy Smoothie

Cayenne pepper is great at easing both arthritis pain as well as headache related pain. Of course, cinnamon and black pepper are known to help as well. The coconut milk and honey help to even out this smoothie a little bit, and tart cherries are known to help with any muscle pain. When put together, this smoothie packs a spicy but powerful pain reliving punch.

Ingredients:

1. 1 Teaspoon Cinnamon Powder
2. ½ Teaspoon Cayenne Pepper Powder
3. ½ Teaspoon Black Pepper, Ground
4. 1 Cup Beet Juice, Chilled
5. ½ Cup Tart Cherries, Pitted & Frozen
6. 2 Tablespoons Honey, Raw
7. 4 Tablespoons Coconut Milk

Directions:

1. Mix everything together, and blend until smooth.

Smoothie #6 Headache & Migraine Smoothie

Magnesium is known to help with headaches and migraines, especially when used as a preventive method. There is no reason to live with migraine pain, and it can severely interrupt your day. Kale is the main star of this smoothie recipe, and it'll help to make sure that your migraines are taken care of.

Ingredients:

1. 1 Teaspoon Flaxseed, Ground
2. 3 Cups Kale, Shredded
3. 1 Medium Banana, Peeled & Frozen
4. 2 Oranges, Peeled & De-seeded
5. 1 Cup Coconut Milk, Frozen

Directions:

1. Mix everything together and blend until smooth.

Chapter 4. Some More Herbal Remedies

There are still many more herbal remedies that you can use if you're looking for quick and effective pain relief, and the best thing is that it's natural. These remedies are easy to use, and they can help you to relax and feel better. There are different types of pain and therefore different remedies, so try to find one that works for you. Many of these herbal remedies can be made in advance.

Remedy #1 Soak for Your Muscles

This soak is a great way to help release tension in your muscles, and it'll also smell wonderful. It can even help you to sleep, and relieve any aches and pains that you may have. Of course, it's recommended for sensitive skin, and any general soreness. It can even help with a stuffy nose.

Ingredients:

1. 1 Tablespoon Sage Leaves
2. 2 Tablespoons Peppermint Leaves
3. 10 Drops Peppermint Essential Oil
4. 2 Tablespoon Pine Needles
5. 1 Tablespoon Juniper Berries
6. ¾ Cup Baking Soda
7. 2 Tablespoons Chamomile Flowers, Dried
8. 2 Cups Epsom Salts

Directions:

1. Take the dry ingredient and wrap them in a cheese cloth, and then tie them. Do not add in the Epsom salts. Mix in the

peppermint essential oil to Epsom salts and store separately.

2. Put in a warm bath, and soak for twenty to thirty minutes to help relieve your aches and pains.

Remedy #2 An Anti-inflammatory Shot

Inflammation often causes pain, such as joint pain, general arthritis, and it can even cause sore muscles. It's important that you make the swelling go down if you want relief from your pain. This is a mixture that should help you to get rid of your inflammation quickly. If you suffer from arthritis or chronic joint pain, you may want to take it once in the morning everyday as a part of your daily routine.

Ingredients:

1. 3 Drops Cinnamon Essential Oil
2. ½ Teaspoon Cloves, Ground
3. ½ Teaspoon Turmeric, Ground
4. ½ Teaspoon Ginger, Ground
5. ½ Teaspoon Honey, Raw
6. 4 Ounces Coconut Milk

Directions:

1. Mix everything together and just take a shot of it every morning. You can do this two to three time's daily if necessary to help keep down inflammation.

Remedy #3 Sore Feet Relief

Pain in the soles of your feet can also cause issues, and it can make it hard for you to get through or even enjoy your day. So it's important to find an easy solution to this type of pain. All you need is mustard seed to relieve foot pain, and it'll help you to feel better quickly. Remember to soak your feet for at least fifteen minutes.

Ingredients:

1.   5 Tablespoons Mustard Seeds, Ground
2.   3 Cups Water

Directions:

1.   Boil the water, and let it cool down. Add in your mustard seed.
2.   Once cool, put into a foot bath to soak your feet in for twenty to thirty minutes. At least soak for fifteen.

Remedy #4 Pain Relieving Ginger Press

This is a great pain relieving compress, and it's easy to make. It even requires only three ingredients. It will help to reduce inflammation, and it'll help you to feel better sooner. Never apply it to an open wound, as it will burn, irritate, and might even cause a mild infection if not cleaned properly or left on too long. It's best to wrap with bandages so that it stays on for the desired time.

Ingredients:

1. 10-15 Slices Ginger, Thin & Peeled
2. 1 Teaspoon Sea Salt, Fine
3. 3-4 Cloves Garlic, Peeled & Crushed

Directions:

1. Take all ingredients and then put them in a mortar and pestle. Crush.
2. Take the pulp and apply it to the sore area, and tape gauze over it. Leave on for six hours, but do not apply it to an open wound as it can case irritation and infection.

Remedy #5 Bath Salts for Pain Relief

This is a bath soak recipe that is great if you want to help yourself sleep while still relieving muscle pains as well as normal aches and pains that may be bothering you. It'll even help to get rid of stress, anxiety, and even depression. You can even make these bath salts up in advance for the perfect soak before you go to bed.

Ingredients:

1. 10 Drops Peppermint Essential Oil
2. 2 Cups Epsom Salts
3. ½ Cup Lavender Buds, Dried
4. 10 Drops Rosemary Essential Oil
5. ½ Cup Chamomile Flowers, Dried

Directions:

1. Add all ingredients into a warm bath. If you don't want the flower buds to go down the drain, then put them in a cheesecloth, tying them in so that they don't get out.
2. Mix everything into the hot water and soak for twenty to thirty minutes. Soaking longer won't hurt. Remember to use warm water for the best results.

Remedy #6 Pain Relieving Lotion Bars

Rub these lotion bars where the pain is. They're better for mild pain, but you can use them on the go. It's easy to package and give as gifts as well. The menthol crystal should be added later on, but you can combine the mango butter, coconut oil, and peppermint together first. These lotions bars are great for a quick but mild relief.

Ingredients:

1. 1/3 Cup Coconut Oil
2. 1/3 Cup Mango Butter
3. 1/3 Cup Beeswax
4. 1 Tablespoon Menthol Crystals
5. 10-12 Drops Peppermint Essential Oil

Directions:

1. Take all the ingredients, ad combine them in a mason jar. Take a saucepan of water, and place the Mason jar into it. The burner should be turned on lower, and the water should simmer. Stir your ingredients until they melt in the jar, and the remove it from heat, stirring in the menthol crystals until they dissolve.
2. Pour into molds, and allow to harden into lotion bars. Any mold will work. Let them cool before popping out. Silicon molds will usually work better.

Remedy #7 Another Joint Pain Shot

Apple cider vinegar can give you a great natural alternative to medicine when trying to relieve joint pain. It helps with chronic inflammation, and honey gives you the antioxidants you need and the sweetness to choke it down when mixed with water.

Ingredients:

1. 2 Tablespoons Apple Cider Vinegar, Raw
2. 2 Tablespoons Honey, Raw
3. 4 Ounces Water, Warm

Directions:

1. Mix everything together and then just drink it down. Do this once every morning if you have chronic joint pain.

Remedy #8 Another Bath or Foot Soak

This is a great pain relieving soak, and it's important that you make it in advance so you can make a relaxing routine out of it. It's easy to make, and it doesn't even require that many ingredients. It's anti-inflammatory, and it's sure to help any muscle pain or chronic inflammation quickly.

Ingredients:

1. 1 Teaspoon Cinnamon, Ground
2. ½ Cup Coconut Oil
3. 1 Cup Epsom Salts
4. 2 Drops Eucalyptus Essential Oil
5. 4 Drops Lavender Essential Oil

Directions:

1. Mix all ingredients together and store in an airtight container until you're ready to use it.

Chapter 5. Salves to Make for Topical Help

There are many salves that you can make to help with pain relief as well, and many of them incorporate different herbs and essential oils. They're easy to make, but they should be made up in advance so that you have them when you need them, since they can be time consuming.

Salve #1 An Overall Warming Salve

A warming salve is great for muscle and joint pain, and that's because the warming sensation helps to relieve the pain you're feeling. Turmeric, ginger, and cayenne powder are all anti-inflammatory, also helping with muscle or joint pain. This is a salve that can even help with nerve pain, but remember to wash your hands before touching your eyes, nose or mouth. Arnica flower are optional, but they are also anti-inflammatory. It can even help with sprains and promotes healing.

Ingredients:

1. ½ Cup Olive Oil
2. ½ Cup Coconut Oil
3. ¼ Cup Beeswax, Grated
4. 1 Tablespoon Cayenne Pepper, Ground
5. 1 Tablespoons Ginger Root, Ground
6. 1 Tablespoons Turmeric Powder
7. 1 Tablespoon Arnica Flowers

Directions:

1. Take the oils, and then put them in a large saucepan. Infuse it with the turmeric, arnica flowers, cayenne powder, and ginger. Let it simmer on low, while stirring occasionally, for

twenty minutes. Strain out the herbs, and then used the infused oil.

2. Put the beeswax into a double boiler, melting it on low, and then add in the infused oil, mixing them together. Spoon into jars for storage, and let cool before sealing and putting up.

Salve #2 For Aches & Pains

This is an everyday pain relief salve, and it's sure to work. It doesn't take that many ingredients, and it's easy to make. Remember that any salve can be time consuming, so always make it in advance, and store it in an airtight container. Keep it in a dark, dry place so that it doesn't lose its potency. You'll need to have an infused oil with St. John's Wort oil already, or you can make it yourself.

Ingredients:

1. ½ Cup St. John's Worth Infused Oil

2. 2 Teaspoons Cayenne Pepper Powder

3. 2 Tablespoons Beeswax, Grated

Directions:

1. Melt the beeswax over a double boiler, and then add in the infused oil and the cayenne powder. Make sure everything is mixed thoroughly, and remove from heat. Pour into different containers to cool before sealing.

Salve #3 Simple Ache Relief

St. John's Wort is great for pain, and so is comfrey leaves. You already know that arnica flowers are anti-inflammatory, and the combination is great for daily aches and pains including chronic pain. It can even help to lessen severe pain, but it's more for mild pain than anything else.

Ingredients:

1. 2 Cups Sweet Almond Oil
2. 3 Ounces Beeswax, Grated
3. ½ Cup St. John's Wort, Dried
4. ½ Cup Comfrey Leaf, Dried
5. ½ Cup Arnica Flowers, Dried

Directions:

1. Take a large saucepan, putting in your oil and all of your dried herbs. Makes sure to turn it to a simmer, and infuse the oil for twenty to thirty minutes.
2. Strain out all of the herbs, while putting the beeswax in a double boiler on low. Let it melt, and then add in the oil.
3. Stir to combine, and move to containers to cool before sealing and storing.

Salve #4 Heating & Numbing Salve

This is usually best for muscles, but it's still good to keep around if you deal with chronic pain. You can use it on any of your muscles, and it takes action fast to give you the relief you need when you need it. It doesn't even have that many ingredients, making it easy to use and easy to make. Clove will help to numb the area, and cayenne provides the heat you need.

Ingredients:

1. 3 Tablespoons Cayenne Infused Oil
2. 10-12 Drops Clove Essential Oil
3. 3 Tablespoons Coconut Oil, Extra Virgin
4. ½ Ounce Beeswax, Grated

Directions:

1. Start by taking three tablespoons of cayenne pepper to a cup of oil if you're making your infused oil. Coconut oil is recommended. Simmer on low in a large

saucepan for thirty minutes, and then strain out the cayenne pepper. Store it on its own, and then take the three tablespoons of the infused oil you need for this recipe, mixing in the clove oil and put it to the side.

2. Take a double boiler, putting in the beeswax and coconut oil. Turn the heat to low, and let both melt, stirring it together.

3. When melted, move it to a bowl and add in your infused oil and clove oil. Mix thoroughly, and put into containers to cool before sealing and storing for later use.

Salve #5 Chronic Pain Salve

This is a great salve for chronic pain, and it'll help to get rid of it quickly and effectively. The wintergreen essential oil helps your chronic pain the most, and the peppermint helps to sooth you when applied topically. Rosemary is meant to help improve circulation, lemongrass helps with muscle tension, and eucalyptus helps because it is anti-inflammatory.

Ingredients:

1. 30 Drops Wintergreen Essential Oil
2. 15 Drops Lemongrass Essential Oil
3. 15 Drops Eucalyptus Essential Oil
4. 15 Drops Rosemary Essential Oil
5. 10 Drops Peppermint Essential Oil
6. 1 ½ Teaspoons Cocoa Butter
7. 3 Teaspoons Beeswax, Grated

Directions:

1. Take the beeswax and cocoa butter, melting over low heat in a double boiler. Make sure to stir so it's blended together, and then take it off the heat to

allow it to cool slightly before adding in your oils.

2. Place into jars to cool before sealing and storing for later use.

Salve #6 Joint & Muscle Pain

This is a great way to help make sure that your joint and muscle pain is a thing of the past, and the clove oil will help to numb the area as well. The peppermint gives a soothing affect, and you have many essential oils with anti-inflammatory effects, which can help with muscle pain and arthritis pain.

Ingredients:

1. 15 Drops Wintergreen Essential Oil
2. 15 Drops Clove Essential Oil
3. 15 Drops Peppermint Essential Oil
4. 15 Drops Rosemary Essential Oil
5. 1 Teaspoon Coconut Oil, Extra Virgin

6. 1 Teaspoon Beeswax, Grated

Directions:

1. Take your coconut oil and beeswax, putting them into a double boiler and melting over low heat. Take off heat, and then add in your essential oils.
2. Spoon into different containers, and then let cool before you let cool.

Salve #7 Lavender Pain Relief

Copaiba oil is a great way to intensify the pain relieving effects of any other oil, and the lavender is soothing and anti-inflammatory. It can even stave off muscle spasms, and marjoram is known to help with arthritis and muscle spasms as well. Add more beeswax if you want a firmer salve.

Ingredients:

1. 6 Drops Copaiba Essential Oils
2. 8 Drops Marjoram Essential Oils
3. 15 Drops Lavender Essential Oil
4. ¼ Cup Coconut Oil, Extra Virgin
5. 1 Teaspoon Beeswax, Grated

Directions:

1. Take a double boiler, putting in your beeswax and coconut oil. Over low heat, melt the two together.
2. Once melted, put it in a small bowl, mixing in all oils until thoroughly blended, and then you can spoon it into different containers to firm up before sealing and storing for later use.

Salve #8 Muscle Pain Relief

You'll find that the copaiba will help to intensify the pain relieving effects of this wonderful salve, but the cypress will help to keep off muscle spasms and relax the tension from your body. So will the marjoram, and when combined it has a powerful soothing effect on your muscles. Just put it wherever you're feeling pain and rub it gently into the muscle.

Ingredients:

1. ¼ Cup Sweet Almond Oil
2. 1 ½ Teaspoons Beeswax, Grated
3. 15 Drops Cypress Essential Oil
4. 4 Drops Copaiba Essential Oil
5. 6-8 Drops Marjoram Essential Oil

Directions:

1. In a double boiler combine your sweet almond oil and beeswax, melting over low heat until combined. Add in essential oils and make sure everything is thoroughly mixed.
2. Take off of heat and put into containers to cool before sealing and storing so that you can use them later.

Chapter 6. Supplements to Bring Relief

There are many supplements that you can use to help you with pain relief as well. Of course, you'll find that you should always tell your doctor before taking a supplement. Any supplement can interact with prescription drugs or over the counter medication, and your doctor can tell you if it is safe for you to take the supplement with anything else that you may already be taking. So make sure that your doctor knows the list of medication you're taking, including over the counter medication.

Supplement #1 Butterbur

This is a supplement that is great for head pain, such as headaches and migraines. If you are experiencing these chronically, then it'll help to make sure that you no longer have to deal with it. It can even help to prevent migraines and headaches, and it stabilizes any irritable blood vessels. It is also very anti-inflammatory.

It's usually fine to take on a regular basis, and it even had the added benefit of helping with joint and arthritis pain of course, it can help with headaches associated with seasonal allergies as well. The dosage will depend on what your doctor thinks that you need, but people take anywhere from seventy-five milligrams twice daily to one hundred milligrams twice daily normally.

Supplement #2 Bromelain

Bromelain is mostly taken for sinus pain, and it's great if you're suffering from anything that is from swelling. It helps with inflammation, and it can help to heal any damaged tissues, including minor bruises. It can relieve sinus congestion and hay fever discomfort as well as sinus infection discomfort. However, you need to be aware that it can thin your blood, and usually it's taken at the sign of symptoms. Its common dosage is two hundred milligrams twice daily, but you usually only take it for four to six days. It is not a supplement that is meant to be taken long term or as a preventative.

Supplement #3 Vitamin D

What most people don't know is that vitamin D is also known to help with pain, especially if you're suffering from back pain. There are many conditions you may be suffering from due to low vitamin D, and it'll often cause lower back pain. You should talk to your doctor to see if vitamin D will help your back pain, and then your doctor will then be able to determine what

type of dosage of vitamin D you should be
taking. It helps with your overall health as well.

Supplement #4 Turmeric

Turmeric is a common supplement that you can usually get ahold of easily, and it's able to help with a lot of pain that is caused by inflammation. Turmeric powder is commonly used in curry and Indian dishes, but when taken as a capsule, you'll find that it can help with stomach upset, swelling, and even joint pain such as arthritis. Just look for your local health store, and usually they'll be carrying turmeric powder. You can ask your doctor for a recommended dosage based on anything else you may be taking, but it's usually safe to follow the instructions on the bottle so long as you have quality turmeric capsules.

Supplement #5 Capsaicin

This is what gives hot peppers the heat that they're known for. It's often used for its medicinal purposes, but you can also use it as a supplement. It has a pain relieving effect when taken, and usually you can find it in a health food store. The relief is short term relief, but you can talk to your doctor about how often it's safe for you to take capsaicin.

Supplement #6 Omega-3 Fatty Acids

It seems like such a simple supplement, but it's known to help with pain. It helps to reduce inflammation, and it also has strong antioxidants which can help with pain. It's easy to get ahold of, and it's safe to take as a preventative method. It'll even help to improve your overall health. It's something that you take daily for the best results, but you still need to let your doctor know that you're taking it.

Supplement #7 Magnesium

Magnesium is also a supplement that is easy to get ahold of, and you'll find it in any health food store. It helps to relax your muscles, and a lot of chronic pain has to deal with you being too tense. It also helps to maximize blood flow. If you have a magnesium deficiency, then you'll find that you'll often get cramps, muscle spasms, and poor blood flow which causes even more pain. It can even cause ailments, so keeping your magnesium levels up will help to keep away chronic pain.

Supplement #8 Devil's Claw

This is a grcat supplement if you're suffering from joint pain, such as arthritis which is commonly caused by inflammation. You should always be careful when taking devil's claw, and it can commonly interact with mediation, so remember to tell your doctor before you start taking it. It's a South African herb, and it helps to reduce overall pain as well. IT can interfere with blood thinners and diabetes medication, however, and should not be taken with these medications.

Supplement #9 Ginger

Ginger is also known to help with arthritis pain and other inflammation related pain. It will not interfere with most medications, and it can help with nausea and an upset stomach. Many people take it with morning sickness or motion sickness, but like any other supplement despite it being a common kitchen spice, you still need to notify your doctor if you plan to take it on a regular basis. Of course, if you don't want to use a ginger supplement, you can add more ginger into your diet. Using fresh ginger is usually best, but you'll find that adding dried ginger will help overtime.

Some Can be Taken Together:

Some supplements actually can be taken together, and they'll help to improve your pain and your overall health. Of course, before mixing supplements that is also something you need to research as well as ask your doctor. Not every supplement can be taken together, just like not every medication can be taken together. Make sure that you know what you're taking, and don't add an over the counter medication to your routine if you haven't gotten it approved by your doctor to be taken with the supplements that you're already taking.

Chapter 7. Essential Oils for Pain Relief

It's not always easy to find pain relief, but you'll find that pain relief can come in essential oil form. You'll find that these blends are great for specific types of pain, but you can use many of the essential oils found in them on their own as well. However, these blends have been crafted to help you with different types of pain so that you know what to use. You can substitute any carrier oil, and when you feel comfortable enough with essential oils, you can even experiment to make your own blends to find the right one to help you.

Some people make blends in advance, but they're quick and easy to make at the spur of the moment as well. If you want to make these essential oils up in advance, you'll want to multiply the recipe and put it in a roller, so that you can roll it onto the area whenever you need to. Just remember to properly label everything you make if you're making it up in advance.

Essential Oil Blend #1 Nerve Pain

Essential oils are a great blend, even with nerve pain. Marjoram essential oil, for example, is great to help with a variety of pains. It helps to relax you and can keep spasms at bay. Lavender essential oil is great with muscle pain and tension, and helichyrsum essential oil is considered to be a potent essential oil for pain relieving effects. It usually helps most with muscle and joint pain, but it can help with nerve pain as well, especially in this essential oil blend.

Ingredients:

1. 3 Drops Helichrysum Essential Oil

2. 2-4 Drops Lavender Essential Oil

3. 2-3 Drops MarjoramEssential Oil

4. 4 Drops Roman Chamomile Essential
    Oil

5. ½ Teaspoon Coconut Oil

Directions:

1. Mix everything together, and then apply
    to the painful area directly. You can do
    this two to three times daily.

Essential Oil Blend #2 General Pain Massage

You really need to massage this oil blend, and
it's a great tonic for nerve pain due to the
lavender essential oil. Rosemary essential oil
will almost use a tingly, and both oils are great
for muscle pain. It can even stop spasming in
its tracks. So make some anytime that you feel

you're having issues with general pain and don't know what it's from.

Ingredients:

1. 2-4 Drops Lavender Essential Oil
2. ½ Teaspoon Coconut Oil, Extra Virgin
3. 5-6 Drops Rosemary Essential Oil

Directions:

1. Mix everything together, and apply it to the area. You can double it for a teaspoon of the blend, and you need to rub it on the place where you're experiencing chronic pain.

Essential Oil #3 Sore Muscle Pain

Any carrier oil can be used with this blend, but sweet almond oil is used because it spreads easily. Feel free to substitute it with another carrier oil if desired. Clove oil is also great for arthritis. Clove oil is actually anti-inflammatory, which can cause muscle pain and arthritis pain. You'll find that it is also a warming oil when peppermint is a cooling oil, so it's a great topical application to relieve any tension you may be feeling.

Ingredients:

1. 1 Teaspoon Sweet Almond Oil
2. 10-12 Drops Peppermint Essential Oil
3. 8-10 Drops Clove Essential Oil

Directions:

1. Mix it all together, and then you can apply it to the area that is causing you issues. It has a warming and cooling effect, which will help to get rid of muscle pain almost instantly.

Essential Oil Blend #4 Arthritis Blend

Rosemary is a muscle relaxant, but it's also great for arthritis. Lavender is also known to help with arthritis, just like tea tree oil. One of the main reason they help is because it helps with inflammation. That's why all three have been blended with a carrier oil, and you can use these oils in larger amounts. Only apply a small amount to the area, and rub it in with circular motions to work it into where it's hurting for quick results.

Ingredients:

1. 1 Teaspoon Olive Oil
2. 5-8 Drops Tea Tree Essential Oil
3. 6-9 Drops Rosemary Essential Oil
4. 10-15 Drops Lavender Essential Oil

Directions:

1. Mix it all together, and apply it to your joints so that you can experience relief quickly.

Essential Oil Blend #5 Back Pain

If you're suffering from chronic pain, you'll often find that back pain is a part of it. You can use any carrier oil you want, but sweet almond oil is most common with back pain because it spreads easily. Lavender is sure to sooth your muscles and help you to let go of tension. The lemon and eucalyptus are great at soothing over your pain as well. Eucalyptus is a warming oil that is great for back pain, spasms, and general muscle aches.

Ingredients:

1. 6 Teaspoons Sweet Almond Oil
2. 4-6 Drops Lavender Essential Oil
3. 1-2 Drops Lemon Essential Oil

4. 2-4 Drops Eucalyptus Essential Oil

Directions:

1. Mix everything together, and then apply
    it to the affected area. Make more as
    needed, and apply when it is needed.

Essential Oil Blend #6 Basic Aches & Pains

Black pepper essential oil is an anti-inflammatory, but it also helps to improve blood flow. These are both reasons that it's a great pain relieving essential oil that has been added into this blend. This blend actually creates a warming effect while helping you to release tension from your body, which will automatically help with your aches and pains.

Ingredients:

1. 4 Drops Black Pepper Essential Oil
2. 3 Drops Lavender Essential Oil
3. 6 Teaspoons Coconut Oil, Extra Virgin
4. 4-6 Drops Roman Chamomile Essential Oil
5. 4 Drops Marjoram Essential Oil

Directions:

1. Mix together and apply gently to the affected area. It's usually best that you rub it in.

Essential Oil Blend #7 Hot Blend

This is a hot blend, and you can use it for arthritis pain or muscle pain, and it'll help you. Of course, the peppermint helps to offset it a little. You can add more or less peppermint essential oil depending on what you feel is best for your skin and your pain. Cinnamon essential oil is great at fighting inflammation as well.

Ingredients:

1. 1 Teaspoon Coconut Oil, Extra Virgin
2. 5-6 Drops Cinnamon Essential Oil
3. 2-3 Drop Peppermint Essential Oil

4. 4 Drops Rosemary Essential Oil

Direction:

1. Just mix everything together and massage it into the painful area. Use circular motions, and you should notice relief quickly.

Essential Oil Blend #8 Pain Number

Clove essential oil is known to numb pain, even when applied topically. Cinnamon essential oil has a slight heating effect which can help to relieve tension, and wintergreen essential oil is known to relieve both muscle and nerve pain, so it helps with a variety of pains in different areas.

Ingredients:

1. 10 Drops Clove Essential Oil

2. 2 Teaspoons Sweet Almond Oil

3. 2 Drops Cinnamon Essential Oil

4. 3-5 Drops Wintergreen Essential Oil

Directions:

1. Mix everything together before applying
    it in circular motions to the affected
    area.

Essential Oil Blend #9 Instant Pain Reducer

Copaiba essential oil is known to strengthen others, and this is an essential oil blend that should bring instant relief. As stated before, the clove essential oil is a great way to numb any pain that you might be feeling, while both the peppermint and wintergreen helps with muscle pain. It keeps this essential oil blend from becoming too hot as well.

Ingredients:

1. 10 Drops Clove Essential Oil
2. 1 Teaspoon Sweet Almond Oil
3. 2-5 Drops Wintergreen Essential Oil
4. 3 Drops Copaiba Essential Oil
5. 5 Drops Peppermint Essential Oil

Directions:

1. Mix all oils together before applying in small circular motions to the affected area.

Essential Oil Blend #10 Anti-inflammatory Relief

This is a blend that has been chosen because of its anti-inflammatory effects, which is what makes it best for arthritis, normal joint, or muscle pain. It can even keep muscles from spasming. All the way from the ginger to the peppermint, it's a soothing essential oil blend that is sure to help. Make sure that your coconut oil is melted before using it. Of course, many people prefer sweet almond oil as a carrier oil in this essential oil blend instead.

Ingredients:

1. 2 Drops ginger Essential Oil
2. 3 Drops Cinnamon Essential Oil

3. 5 Drops Rosemary Essential Oil

4. 2 Teaspoons Coconut Oil

5. 2 Drops Black Pepper Essential Oil

6. 4 Drops Peppermint Essential Oil

Directions:

1. Mix all oils together before applying to the affected area. This oil works best, like most blends, when it's been rubbed in gently.

Chapter 8. Bonus Tips for Pain Relief

There are still many things you can do to manage your pain, and the tips found in this chapter will help you to cope with it in a healthy and natural way. You don't need to let pain rule your life, and you certainly don't have to put up with pain on a regular basis. Instead, you're going to need to make sure that you use the remedies provided in this book and the tips to help keep your pain at manageable levels if not completely eased.

Tip #1 Avoid Inflammation Causing Food

Most chronic pain is caused by chronic inflammation, and you can avoid inflammation causing foods if you want to help get rid of it.

Otherwise, it's counterproductive to try to get rid of it with herbal and natural remedies. Some inflammation causing foods dairy, chocolate, citrus fruits, high-fat red meat, processed foods, coffee, soda, and even wheat products. Of course, you can't have eggplant or tomatoes or other nightshade vegetables if you want to keep the inflammation at bay. Having an inflammation reducing diet is much more likely to help you deal with your chronic pain.

Tip #2 Get a Massage

Often, chronic pain is a result of your muscles being too tense. Getting a massage can really help. A professional massage will usually help the most, but having someone that you love and cares about you will help as well. This will help you to relax and keep your muscles from tensing, which will only make your pain worse. This is especially good for back, neck, and leg pain. If its neck and leg pain you can even gently massage the area yourself.

Tip #3 Reduce Your Stress

Reducing your stress won't get rid of chronic pain, but it'll help to lessen it. This is because the stress in our life actually intensifies chronic pain, and it can cause you to feel overwhelmed and anxious as well, which will continue the cycle. There are many ways to reduce your stress. Listening to music can help because it uplifts your mood, and you can even take relaxing meditation, yoga, or use progressive muscle relaxation. It's important to relax before bed if you want to help lessen some of your stress.

Tip #4 Exercise Regularly

When you exercise you release endorphins, which are chemicals in your brain which will help to block pain signals and even improve your mood. So it helps with pain, stress, and even anxiety. It even helps to strengthen your muscles, which can have a pain reducing effect as well. It also has the added benefit of helping to control blood sugar levels, help you lose weight and keep a reasonable weight, and reduces your risk of developing heart disease.

Tip #5 Use Positive Imagery

If you want to relax quickly and manage your pain, you often need to think about something else. Dwelling on pain only makes it worse, so while you're waiting for an herbal remedy to kick in, try using some positively imagery. Think of a place that really makes you happy, and try to imagine every detail of that place. Pull it up as vividly as you can in your mind as you possibly can. Try to pull up every sensory detail, and this will help to make the experience a little more real for you. This will help to transport you into a happier place while you try and sort through your pain or wait for something to help it.

Remember It Takes Time:

What you should always keep in mind is that it takes time to handle your pain. You'll never find a miracle solution, not even a cream. You need to look for what really works for you, and always take into account what type of pain you might be experiencing. If you're trying to treat the wrong pain, then you won't find much relief in anything. Try out different teas, supplements, bath soaks, or salves if you want to find what really works best for you.

Ask your doctor to see if they can help you to figure out what type of pain you're experiencing, and this will help you to narrow down on what type of pain you should be trying to treat. You can even ask what they think about adding in certain teas, supplements, or habits to your routine to increase your health and the way you manage your pain naturally.

www.ingramcontent.com/pod-product-compliance
Lightning Source LLC
Chambersburg PA
CBHW061751050726
47598CB00002B/700